THE OMAD WORKOUT

*How You Can Exercise and Get Fit on the
One Meal A Day Intermittent Fasting Diet*

MARKUS WILKINSEN

Legal Notes

monetary loss due to the information herein, either directly or indirectly. This disclaimer applies to any loss, damages or injury caused by the use and application, whether directly or indirectly, of any advice or information presented, whether for breach of contract, tort, negligence, personal injury, criminal intent, or under any other cause of action.

You agree to accept all risks of using the information presented inside this book.

Permission is not granted to reproduce, duplicate, or transmit any part of this document in electronic or printed format. Recording of this publication is also prohibited and storage of this document is not allowed without the written permission from the publisher.

Table of Contents

INTRODUCTION

When looking to lose weight, the two most common areas people look at is their diet, and their fitness. Hitting the gym is a good place to start but understandably, the idea of spending hours at the gym can be deterring to some people. We all have 24 hours a day with our own responsibilities, obligations, and priorities. Our jobs, our families, our children, and our friends all clamor for attention and our time, and some of us choose to take on additional responsibilities like volunteering or getting involved in local communities.

It is no wonder that amidst all the hustle and bustle of our lives, the gym is also one of the first things we put off or drop from our schedules altogether.

After all, exercise is 50% of the equation. Our diet is the other 50% and it controls the calories we eat and if we consume less energy than we expand we lose weight. It sounds simple right? We can cut 300 kcal of energy by running three miles or we can stop ourselves from eating a bar of chocolate that we would normally eat.

Between the two, not eating the chocolate bar sounds like an easier choice to make.

However, if you want not only to maximize your weight loss but to be healthy, then exercise is what you need. The secret is simple: be as efficient as possible with both your exercise and your diet.

In the first part of this book, we will look at the exercise portion of the equation. In addition to cardiovascular exercises like running, walking, and cycling you should perform some strength training exercises will help you burn more calories by raising your resting metabolic rate.

The secret to weight loss with exercise is to adopt an effective exercise routine that complements your diet. When your exercise routine and your diet work together, you don't have to spend hours at the gym a few times a week to shed a few pounds and get yourself into shape. As you can tell from the title of this book, you just need to work out while eating One Meal a Day (OMAD).

The OMAD diet would cover the second part of the book. With your diet, it should be easy to follow and satisfy you. Most dieters fail due to what is known as yo-yo dieting where people end up putting on the weight they have lost after achieving their goals. This is common because the diet that they have put themselves on is not something that they can sustain in the long run.

The One Meal a Day (OMAD) Diet is a weight loss method based on intermittent fasting, meal frequency, and meal timing. It is a way to lose fat and keep it off while eating whatever you want.

This is not a fad diet, nor is it a temporary weight loss solution. A short term diet is unhealthy and will increase your weight when you stop the diet, indeed many dieters have experienced a yo-yo effect on their weight. They do not lose enough weight to be satisfied and end up giving up their diet.

Before we go any further, I would like to make it clear that this book is not a substitute for professional medical advice. Your health is of the utmost importance and you must consult a doctor before changing your diet, especially if you have a history of medical or dietary problems. Also, when exercising, having a trainer will help to minimize the risk of injury.

Diet or Exercise - Which Comes First?

When starting out on your weight loss journey, a common question that I hear is "which comes first, should I start with diet or exercise?"

To answer this question the Stanford University School of Medicine conducted a study with 200 participants who were initially inactive in 2013. What they did was separate the participants into four groups:

1. The first group was counseled to adjust their diet and begin exercising immediately.

2. The second group was counseled to adjust their diet immediately, then work on adding an exercise routine.

3. The third group was counseled to begin an exercise routine immediately, then work on adjusting their diet.

4. The last group was a control group and did not make any changes.

The participants in this study were advised to follow the US National Fitness and Nutrition Requirements. These requirements are 150 minutes of weekly exercise, and five to nine servings of fruit and vegetables daily. In addition, saturated fats should be limited to a maximum of 10%.

What they found was very interesting:

- The participants who started dieting and exercise at the same time expectedly had the best results and were best able to stick to the recommended diet and exercise.

- Those that started exercising first before starting on their diet also managed to stick to the recommended diet and exercise but not as well as the first group.

- However, the participants who started the diet before exercising only managed to meet the dietary goals, and failed to meet the exercise goals.

When starting dietary changes, people get engrossed with the diet and are less able to motivate themselves to exercise. On the flip side, starting with exercise allows people to see a visible change in their bodies. This motivates them further to stick with their dietary and fitness changes.

Focusing on a diet change first actually interferes with establishing an exercise routine. So ideally you should begin with both at the same time or less ideally if you don't have the time or energy to make both changes, start with exercise.

CHAPTER 1

Understanding Fitness and Weight Loss

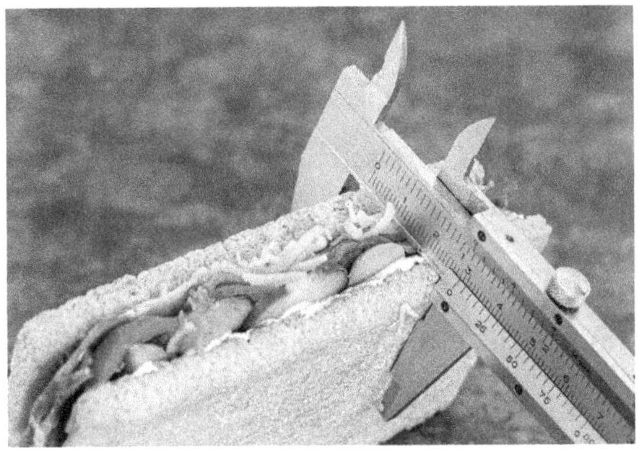

When you are starting out on your diet and exercise routine, you will naturally have many questions about what to expect. This chapter is dedicated to prepare you for the exercise portion of your new routine.

Weight Loss vs. Fat Loss

While dieting and working out, most people do not realize that there are many differences between losing weight, and losing fat.

When we lose weight, the weight that we lose can come from either essential or non-essential sources. For example, losing weight due to losing blood may not be a good thing, but losing weight from going to the bathroom may be normal. Weight loss can also come from perspiration, dehydration, diet, and exercise.

To ensure that the weight we lose is permanent and healthy, we need to lose fat. Fat is the adipose tissue that our bodies store for when food is unavailable and it needs energy to carry out our bodily processes. We need energy to live, and when there is no food our bodies turn to fat.

When we lose fat, it is typically through exercise and diet. However, fat loss and weight loss do not always happen together as we will see in the next section. This may not always be a bad thing.

Fat Loss Through Diet

When you have a highly nutritious diet with lots of protein, fat, fresh fruits, vegetables, complex carbohydrates, and nuts you will start to lose fat. These foods are low in sugar and any carbohydrates you consume are complex carbs. This will prevent spikes in your insulin levels, and when coupled with fasting (like on the OMAD diet), you will end up burning fat.

The 20 hour fasting window will put your body into ketosis, which is where your body consumes ketones produced from the fat stores in your liver instead of relying on blood glucose as a source of energy.

Once your body reaches a healthy body fat percentage it begins to use the nutrition it receives to power your body and stops storing fat like it previously did. The healthy body fat percentage is between 10% to 25% in men and 20% to 30% in women,

Fat Loss Through Exercise

Everything we do requires a surprising amount of energy, even simple tasks like walking, or carrying groceries. What more when we push our bodies with exercise?

When we work out we engage our body's energy expenditure processes, and this includes the use of our stored adipose (fat) tissues. This makes exercise or sports very effective fat loss methods because they work on two levels; by burning fat and creating tears in our muscles, which encourages it to grow.

When your muscles are damaged during exercise, this is a natural process which forces your body to use calories from food and stored fat to fuel the repair process which is how your muscles grow and how we become stronger. When doing so, your body continues to use up adipose tissue well after your work out.

Muscle is also more metabolically active than fat meaning that it burns more calories when we are at rest as compared to fat. It is estimated that muscle tissue will burn about 10 calories per pound each day, as compared to fat that burns up to three calories per pound.

Fat vs. Muscle Weight

When we start out on dieting and exercise, a common objective is to lose weight. What they often overlook is that gaining muscle will offset any fat loss at least at the beginning. Our bodies are great at adapting to changes in our diet. When we change our calorie intake we will see more weight loss in the first few weeks, but as our bodies adapt to the diet the weight loss will naturally slow down.

Also, as we exercise, we may end up putting on some of the weight that we have shed. That is because muscle tissue is denser than fat. As you begin to lose fat and put on muscle you will see that your clothing may drop a size but your weight will not change much.

However, having more muscle and less fat is beneficial to your overall health despite not losing weight. When you have less fat in your body, you lower your risk for obesity related diseases such as diabetes, hypertension, and heart diseases.

Training Frequency

When you are trying to lose fat and gain muscle it is best to have a schedule. That way your fitness becomes a priority and you will set aside time for working out.

There are many ways that people schedule their training from splitting each day by muscle groups, focusing on one muscle group a day, to splitting their workout into upper/lower body sessions, or just committing to working out three times a week. The idea here is that you must let your muscles recover from a workout before stressing it again.

Mentally has the additional benefit of making your work outs more relaxing as you do not always have to do high intensity, heart pumping, muscle straining exercises when you are feeling sore.

Rest Days and Muscle Recovery

When it comes to muscle building, it is actually your rest days that grow your muscles, not your time at the gym.

When you are exercising, your recovery is just as important as your work outs. Some trainers would argue that it is even more important as without rest your body will not recover from the stress of exercise and your muscles will not grow.

Regardless of whether you're lifting weights, running, or doing bodyweight exercises, you damage your muscle fibers and create tears in the muscles. This is normal as your muscles break down to perform physical activity.

When at rest, your muscles start to repair themselves and strengthen. This leads to larger muscles and correspondingly an increase in strength. However, muscle soreness was found to peak 48 hours after exercise therefore leading some trainers to recommend at least 72 hours of rest between training sessions but this could vary depending on your physiology, age, and diet.

CHAPTER 2

The Science of Fasting and Working Out

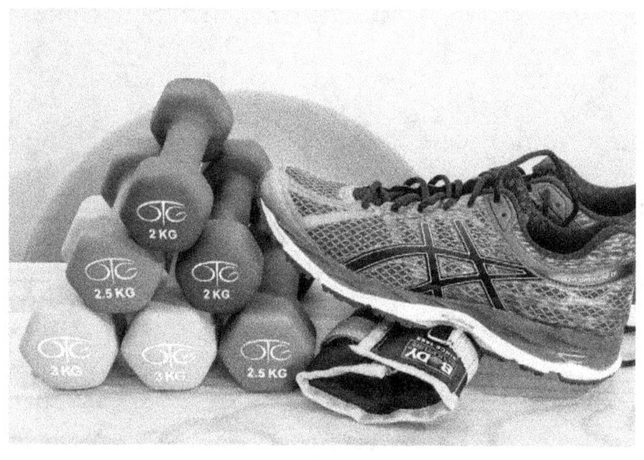

There are a lot of beliefs regarding exercising in a fasted state. There is "common wisdom" that exercising in a fasted state will cause you to lose more muscle than fat, or that eating before exercise can spike your blood sugar which would affect your performance. There are arguments both for and against exercising on an empty stomach.

So should you or should you not exercise in a fasted state?

The short answer is that working out while hungry will help boost your fat-burning potential during exercise.

Benefits of Exercising in a Fasted State

The University of Bath die a study on meal timing and physical activity in 2017, and they have found that exercising on an empty stomach improves the long term effects of exercise on our lipid, insulin, and blood sugar.

Exercise is more effective in a fasted state for two reasons.

Firstly, fasting can trigger a dramatic rise in human growth hormone (HGH), this is also known as "the fitness hormone." HGH is also secreted when we are asleep and is believed to help with anti-aging as the amount our bodies produce decreases as we age.

More importantly, HGH can also increase our muscle growth and improve exercise performance. Fasting helps you to burn body fat which increases HGH production, and it lowers insulin levels which research has shown to disrupt HGH production. After fasting for three days HGH levels can increase by up to 300%, and after a week it can increase by up to 1,250%.

Secondly, exercise coupled with the lack of food triggers our bodies sympathetic nervous system. This forces our bodies to break down the fat and glycogen that it stores, meaning we are more effective at burning fat while fasted.

When exercising in a fasted state, our bodies burn off the stored sugar and then starts to work on the fat we have stored, converting it into ketones for fuel.

There are many studies that have shown that exercising in a fasted state increases fat loss by up to 20 percent. This is because when we are not fasted, insulin is increased in our body, and higher insulin levels are linked with a slow-down of fat burning metabolism by the same amount of approximately 20 percent.

This basically means that exercising on an empty stomach makes our bodies more efficient at using fat rather than sugar as fuel giving us a better result for our effort. This is the reason that so many soldiers and marines exercise before their breakfast.

What Happens When You Fast and Exercise?

As we discussed in an earlier chapter, the Standford University School of Medicine has shown that diet and exercise have a synergistic relationship; they both help your weight loss. Diet restricts your caloric intake and increases your intake of valuable nutrients, and exercise helps to burn calories as well as build lean muscle mass. Building muscle will help to burn more calories while at rest.

On the OMAD diet, when we are in a fasted state our bodies start to use our stored fat and glycogen reserves as its main energy source to provide energy for our daily activities.

But what about when you exercise while you are in a fasted state?

A 2009 study showed that carbohydrate restriction through intermittent fasting, when coupled with exercise, can increase the endurance among trained athletes.

Exercising with low glycogen in our bodies also increases the mitochondrial biogenesis, which is the process wherein new mitochondria are formed within the cells. Mitochondria provide more energy to sustain individual cells during the workout and are known as the powerhouse of the cell.

Lastly, when working in a fasted state, the preservation mechanism of the body that protects active muscles are activated. This prevents active muscles from wasting away, which is known as muscle atrophy. Therefore, we are effectively burning our fat and glycogen stores instead of muscles contrary to popular belief.

Remember those exercise routines burn energy that supports weight loss and training under a fasted state provides some unique benefits in terms of fat loss.

Does It Affect Men and Women Differently?

Men and women have different physiologies. Therefore it is important to consider this when deciding on your workout routines during your fasting periods.

The effects of fasting among men and women are almost the same with regard to glucose and insulin response. However, Monica Klempel a researcher at the University of Illinois found that due to the menstrual cycles of women longer periods of fasting resulted in significant metabolic responses.

This includes increased production of cortisol and a disrupted circadian clock, both of which are signs of stress. In addition, there was found to be a huge reduction of LDL (good cholesterol) levels among women who maintained an intermittent fasting diet for a sustained period of time.

Dr Bajaj, the Director and Head of Medicine at the Motilal Nehru College in India has also linked prolonged fasting to early onset menopause, stress, and reproductive health issues.

But this does not mean that the OMAD diet is dangerous to women. It is important to take note that the dangerous effects of fasting among women were observed on longer and sustained fasting periods. Therefore it is important that the fasting window should be less than 24 hours, and women should discontinue fasting if pregnant, stressed, or unable to adapt to the new lifestyle.

It is important to take note that while men do not have a problem losing weight and burning off fat, it might take longer for women to see the same amount of fat being burned from their bodies. Women should attempt to approach the OMAD diet differently; their focus should be on the quality of the food that they eat, exercising regularly, and getting more sleep.

While men and women will have different experiences, they can both find effectiveness in working out on the OMAD diet.

CHAPTER 3

How to Create Your Workout Plan

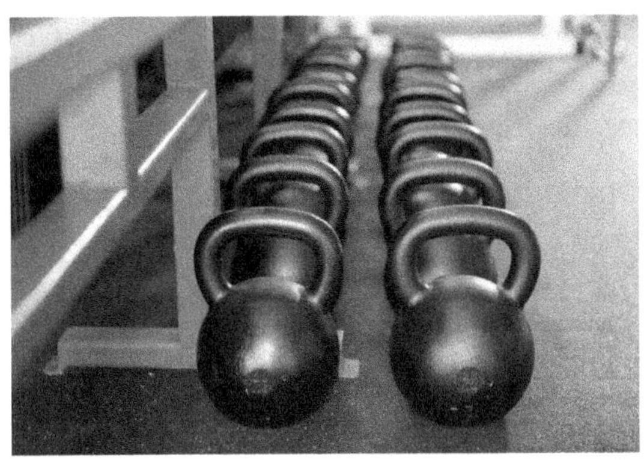

Just diet alone is insufficient for a healthy lifestyle or permanent weight or fat loss. It is important that we incorporate exercise into our routine to help our bodies shed off the excess pounds as well as to build muscle.

The challenge, however, with exercising while on the OMAD diet is that people worry that they would not have enough energy to perform their daily activities, let alone exercise. Conditioning is essential when on the OMAD diet. If you have already been exercising regularly, you would have noticed that your body burns off fat and raises your metabolism up.

When creating your workout plan may be a straightforward matter. But if you are on the OMAD diet and are frequently in a fasted state, there are additional things you would need to take into consideration. If not done properly, you may end up injuring yourself or doing harm to your body. Working out with an empty stomach should be done correctly so that you don't lose your muscle mass.

This chapter will cover the things that you need to know in order to create a good plan and exercise safely on the OMAD diet.

Start with Assessing Yourself

When you are starting out, whether it is with the OMAD diet, exercise, or both, you should start with assessing your situation. Comparing yourself to others may not be realistic, and if you are just starting out it can be downright discouraging, so then how should you assess your fitness?

One way is to see a doctor for a full assessment. This is a great option if you have leg or knee problems and intend to do high impact exercises like running, or if you have back injuries or other injuries that may affect your exercise and fitness.

Another way is to do a standardized assessment like running a mile and timing yourself or doing the CrossFit "Baseline" workout of the day (WOD). These standardized assessments can be used to benchmark yourself at regular intervals and track your progress as you improve in your fitness.

Understanding how healthy and fit you are will help you to set your expectations and goals, and help to ensure that your workout plan is suitable and realistic for you. It is also a way for you to measure your improvements over time.

The other thing you should look at is your availability. How much time can you commit? How much time do you want to commit? Remember that we all have our priorities, so you would have to set yours.

Even if it's just an hour or thirty minutes, if you fully dedicate yourself to your workout, it is better than nothing. If you plan it right, you can accomplish a lot in the time you have allocated.

Timing Your High and Low Intensity Exercises

This is the key to structuring your workouts while following the OMAD diet.

Schedule your low intensity cardio exercises during fasting periods

A low intensity cardio exercise is different for everyone as it depends on their fitness levels. Generally, you should be able to have a conversation without running out of breath while doing this exercise.

Walking, cycling, or doing simple bodyweight exercises as well as exercises that isolate and train one muscle group. These will help you to burn more fat with simple movements while minimizing the risk of you feeling dizzy.

Schedule your high intensity workouts after your meal

High intensity workouts are the ones that leave you sweaty and panting. As the name implies, they are fast paced and gets your heart pumping. To maximize fat loss, high intensity workouts should be scheduled after meals. After you have eaten, your body has glycogen that can be used as fuel.

It is recommended that you do 2 to 3 high intensity workouts during the week.

Deciding Your Workout Schedule

When you are trying to create your working routine and set a schedule, there are many things that you need to consider such as your age, biology, diet, goals, and your time available. In addition, when on the OMAD diet you will also need to consider your meal window.

If you are just starting out on the OMAD diet and working out it is crucial to determine your current situation. How much time you can dedicate for exercise and especially consider when those timings are in relation to your meal window timing.

Generally, on the OMAD diet, your fast should last 18 to 20 hours, which would take you through the night. Most people on OMAD have their meal window in the afternoon or early evening which would give them some time to schedule a workout session before their meal. Depending on your preference, if you break your fast in the morning or early afternoon you will need to adjust your routine accordingly.

Waiting for the eating window to open may be difficult enough for some people, and having to wait for it after working out only makes it much tougher. Remember that your body needs to refuel after an intense work out.

Instead, I would suggest you consider scheduling your workout two hours or two and a half hours before your meal. Try to keep an hour between the end of your workout and the start of your meal as this is when experts believe is the post-exercise anabolic window.

The theory is that consuming nutrients an hour after exercise is supposed to be more effective at rebuilding muscle tissue and restoring energy.

Maximizing Your Workout

When looking to create your workout schedule and maximize the benefit with a limited amount of time, there are several things that you need to take into consideration.

Warm up exercises

Before starting your workout exercises you should warm up by doing static and dynamic stretching exercises. The purpose of doing these warm up exercises is to get your blood flowing and slowly raise your heart rate and breathing rate, which would help you to avoid injuries later.

Static stretching involves holding a position for 30 seconds or more to stretch the muscle while a dynamic warm up involves stretching through a range of motion.

Some examples of dynamic stretching are squats, jumping jacks, and lunges.

Select one exercise for each big muscle groups:

There are 5 major muscle groups which are the chest, abdominals, legs, arms, and back. (covered in Chapter 4), and you need to ensure that your workout plan has one exercise for each muscle group.

Perform 3 to 5 sets for each exercise

To get the most out of your workout and ensure it is effective you should perform 3 to 5 sets for each exercise with at least 10 reps per set. If you are unable to reach this number, you should slowly work your way up to 10 reps.

Diversify your workouts

You can select a different exercise for each muscle group to switch it up and keep it diversified. This keeps your workouts more interesting.

Do alternating sets or circuits

An alternating set is when you select two exercises that work the same muscle group, and you do those with a short rest between each set.

A circuit is a set of exercises that you perform one after the other, usually with a rest in between. Each exercise would work a different muscle group.

Always keep your workout short

Exercising for a longer period does not make your training more effective and may be counterproductive. The ideal exercise length should be an hour at most, which is enough for 25 minutes of cardio, and 25 minutes of muscle building exercise. Remember that you should also dedicate 5 minutes before and after to warm up and cool down your muscles to avoid injuries.

Stretch after working out

Stretching after exercise is very important as it helps improve your flexibility as well as your range of motion.

It also reduces the risk of injury, particularly on the connective tissues of your muscles.

Moreover, it is also a great way to relieve the physical stress of exercising, as it can reduce lactic acid formation. This is what causes soreness of the muscles that you will be familiar with a few hours after exercise.

CHAPTER 4

Preventing Injuries During Your Work Out

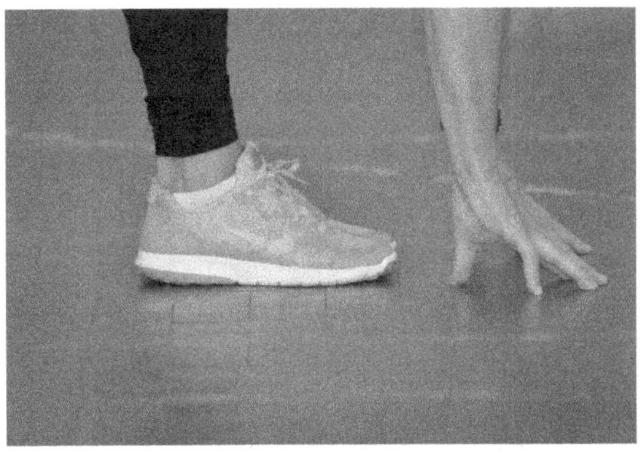

Regardless of whether you're a beginner or a pro, every person that exercises is concerned about injuries. A minor sprain may be inconvenient and affect your quality of life for a few days but anything more serious and you may lose all motivation to exercise for a long, long time.

It is therefore your responsibility to ensure that you take precautions as much as possible to prevent injuries from happening and keeping you away from your weight loss and fitness goals.

Preventing Muscle Cramps

Everyone will experience a muscle cramp. It is the sudden tightening of your muscles and it stops you in your tracks. It usually happens on your calves, but it can also happen on your lower back, abdomen, and other places where you have muscles.

Though they are generally harmless it will put a stop to your work out for at least the next few minutes. Not to mention they are also painful and uncomfortable. But what causes muscle cramps in the first place?

A muscle cramp is commonly caused by one of three things: the overuse of a muscle, strain in the muscles, or dehydration.

Less commonly, it could be due to a medical condition or a lack of minerals in your diet such as potassium, calcium, or magnesium.

To prevent a muscle cramp, you should warm up your muscles. If you are just starting exercise, you may need to take a longer period to warm up but it will be worth it if it keeps your joints flexible.

Also, you should keep your body well hydrated. If you are working out under the sun, or doing high intensity exercise cramping is more likely to occur as you are at a higher risk of dehydration.

Hydration has additional benefits which we will cover in the next section.

If you do get a muscle cramp during your exercise, understand that this is normal and will most likely go away in just a few minutes. However, you may be feeling sore a bit longer. Sit down, take a breath, and take this opportunity to hydrate yourself. You should also gently stretch the muscle, slowly at first to help loosen up the muscles. You can also gently massage the affected muscle.

The Importance of Hydration

Staying hydrated is important at all times, but it is especially important when fasting as well as before and after exercise. Since our bodies are up to 65 percent water, and our brains are 75 percent water, failing to stay hydrated could damage our bodies.

Your body will not function properly without adequate water, as it is needed to carry out its everyday processes. In fact, your body needs pure water more than it needs daily food, as you can go without food for much longer than you can go without water. We depend on water for our survival.

In one hour of exercise the body can lose more than a quarter of its water. Dehydration leads to muscle fatigue and loss of coordination. Without an adequate supply of water the body will lack energy and muscles may cramp. So, drink before, during and after a workout.

Lean muscle tissue contains more than 75 percent water, so when the body is short on H_2O, muscles are more easily fatigued. Staying hydrated helps prevent the decline in performance, strength, power, aerobic and anaerobic capacity during exercise. So, when your muscles feel too tired to finish a workout, grab a drink of water before getting back to it.

The Importance of Warming Up

Before starting on your exercise routine, it is highly advised for you to warm up by doing some stretching exercises. This is also an excellent time for you to adjust your mindset, clear your thoughts, and get yourself emotionally pumped to work out.

Additionally, warming up provides you with several benefits such as:

It improves your flexibility and range of motion

As we stretch our muscles during warm up, our muscles and tendons will lengthen which will help to extend the range of your movement. This allows your joints to move more freely making your arms and legs more flexible.

It improves muscle performance

As your range of movement increases, you will find that exercise becomes easier. You are able to sustain longer work outs without feeling exhausted and you will find that your performance increases.

It helps to prevent injuries

When your muscles and tendons are well flexed and in warmed up properly, they will be able to take on more stress. You can exercise harder and for a longer period with less likelihood of injury.

It reduces muscle tension

If you perform regular warm up exercises, it is less likely for your muscles to constrict. This will definitely relieve you of any muscle pain or problems, and prevent muscle cramps. You will also experience less soreness after exercise.

CHAPTER 5

Training The Major Muscle Groups

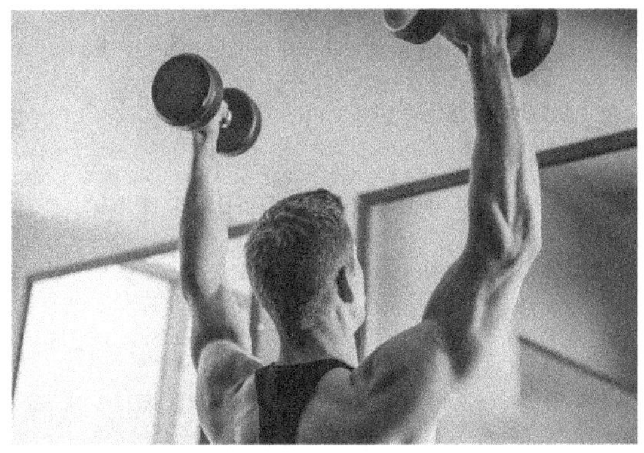

The human body has over 600 muscles which make up about 40% of your body weight. These muscles are what contracts and flexes, and are used for any sort of movement whether we are lifting bags of groceries, running for the bus, or typing on a keyboard.

However, deciding which muscle groups to train together can be confusing as a simple search on the internet would tell you. There are different trainers with many different opinions. Some believe that they should be grouped by activity such as the chest and triceps, which are used with bench pressing and overhead pressing. Others believe that they should be separated so it isolates each muscle group for maximum effectiveness.

So, how are you supposed to put all of this into an effective training routine?

All you want is a program that helps you add muscle to all the right places without requiring you to be at the gym for a few hours regularly. In this chapter I will show you how to work all your muscle groups in an hour.

When you are working out and trying to build muscle, knowing the right kind of exercises in every muscle group allows you to focus on each muscle group one at a time. This allows you to minimize injuries, prevent muscle imbalances, and build your muscles faster.

The major muscle groups are:

1. Chest

2. Back

3. Arms & Shoulders

4. Legs & Glutes

5. Abdominals (Abs)

In the next section, we will look at each of these groups and discuss the muscles as well as some exercises you can do to build the muscles in each group. With each section, there are some exercises that are bodyweight exercises meaning that you can do them without the use of gym equipment.

If you are unsure of how to perform these exercises, please consult with a personal trainer to avoid any injury or harm to yourself.

Muscle Group 1

The first major muscle group is the chest, and the main muscle group of the chest is the pectorals, also known as the "pecs" major. The chest is divided into two parts, pectoralis major, and pectoralis minor.

The pectorals or pecs are the large chest muscles. They are full of thick muscle fibers and add size to the upper body. While it does improve your physique, these muscles are used throughout the day. The main function of this muscle group is to provide support when you hold objects in front of your body and they are activated when you reach across your body.

Putting on a seat belt, combing your hair, or reaching into your back pocket are simple everyday activities that use your pectoral muscles.

To train your chest, you can do the following exercises:

- Push ups
- Bench Presses
- Chest Flies

Muscle Group 2

The second major muscle group is the back, and it is the most complex major muscular structure in the human body. It is a combination of 5 muscles that starts from above the glutes (buttocks) and goes until the neck and shoulders.

These muscles work together and complement each other to enable us to stand, reach out our arms, and pull things towards us.

The 5 muscles of the back are:

Latissimus Dorsi

The Latissimus Dorsi is also known as the "lats" or "wings" and is one of the first muscles that come to mind when discussing back muscles. A pronounced Lattisimus Dorsi has a pronounced "V" shape because of the protruding muscles under the arms and behind the ribs.

The lats enable your body to pull and compliment the arms. When you reach up and grab something off a shelf or when swimming, your lats are one of the main muscles used.

To train your lats you can do:

- Pull Ups
- Dead Lifts
- Barbell Rows

Rhomboid

The rhomboids are located in the upper back, underneath the trapezius. They not visible from outside and originate from the spinal cord and merge into the scapular bone. While these muscles cannot be seen, they strengthen the scapulae when you bring your shoulders together.

To train your Rhomboid muscles you can do:

- Pull Ups
- Barbell Rows

Trapezius

The Trapezius is also known commonly known as "traps", that are located between shoulders and the neck. The traps are a complex set of muscles and consists of upper, middle, and lower traps which extends to the lower back.

The traps control the shoulder blades (scapulae) and come into play when shrugging or moving your neck, and they provide support when you lift item above your head.

To train your Traps you can do:

- Shrugs

- Deadlifts

- Barbell Rows

Teres Major

This muscle lies underneath the lat, and it is a small but important muscle of the back. It is sometimes called the "little lat", as it works in conjunction with the lats, but also with the rotator cuff muscles.

While the teres major is usually worked in conjunction with the lats, if you want to train your teres major you can do:

- Dumbbell Pullovers

Alternatively, you can train this muscle whenever you do:

- Deadlifts

- Shoulder Presses

- Barbell Rows

Erector Spinae

The erector spinae or spinal erectors is a set of muscles that line your spinal column from your lower back to the upper back.

These muscles allow you to straighten and rotate the back and are key to maintaining a good posture. They are also important when bending your body forward, and sideways. When well developed, good erector spinae muscles will give a boost to your total strength.

To train your erector spinae muscles you can do:

- Deadlifts

- Squats

Muscle Group 3

The third major muscle group is the arms, and they are used when you use your arms or hands. They are used for four major types of movement which are: flexion, extension, abduction, adduction.

Biceps

The biceps are at the front of your upper arm and they control the motion of the shoulder, elbow, and forearm. The biceps are one of the most popular muscle group for bodybuilders, powerlifters, and especially to guys new to the gym.

The biceps are essential in lifting, especially when bending or curling the arm towards your body.

To train your biceps you can do:

- Barbell Curls
- Reverse Grip Curls
- Pull Ups

Triceps

The triceps are muscles in the back of the upper arm, behind the biceps. These muscles help to stabilize the shoulder joint and are used when the elbow joint to be straightened. Common, everyday activities that use your triceps are pushing, pulling, and using a pen.

To train your triceps you can do:

- Bench Presses

- Tricep Extensions

- Dips

Deltoids

The deltoids, or delts, are the shoulder muscles located above the biceps and have a triangular shape. They consist of 3 parts: anterior deltoid, medial deltoid, and posterior deltoid.

The deltoids are used when we flex our shoulders and help to provide support when we carry things such as groceries. When our arms are extended the deltoids help to keep our grocery bags away from our knees and thighs.

To train your deltoids you can do:

- Overhead Presses

- Shoulder Presses

Muscle Group 4

The fourth muscle group is comprised of your leg and glutes (also known more commonly as your buttocks). These muscles are one of the main workhorses of your body and you use them all the time whenever you are standing, walking, or otherwise moving around. Your leg and glutes help to hold your body up and keep your body balanced.

Gluteals

The glutes are the largest muscles in your body and form the muscles of your buttocks. These muscles help with movements of the hips and thighs, and they are key muscles that you use to move your legs especially backwards and sideways. The glutes also help you maintain balance in walking or running.

To train your glutes you can do:

- Squats
- Side Skates
- Hip Thrusts

While there are gym machines and weights to train your glutes, bodyweight training exercises have been shown to be more effective as weight machines may isolate only a single layer of your glute muscles.

Hamstrings

The hamstrings are the huge muscle group behind your thighs. These muscles help to flex your knee joints and extend your thighs behind your body. Whenever you are walking, running, or jumping, your hamstrings are being used to move your body forward by flexing. Note that the hamstrings are stretched when you are in a sitting position, so prolong periods of sitting may affect your hamstrings.

To train your hamstrings you can do:

- Romanian Deadlifts

- Squats

Quadriceps

The quadriceps (also known as "quads") are the four muscles at the front of your thighs and consists of four separate muscles originating from the femur bone and attach to your kneecaps. These muscles help in extending the knee and are used for walking, running, and jumping. The quadriceps is the second largest major muscular structure in the human body after the back.

To train your quads you can do:

- Squats

- Rope Skipping

- Lunges

Gastrocnemius

The gastrocnemius is a fancy name for your calf muscles, which are at the back of your lower legs. These muscles are used to move the heel and your feet and are used mainly when walking, running, jumping, and climbing up stairs.

To train your calves you can do:

- Calf Raises

- Ankle Circles

- Balance Boards

Muscle Group 5

The fifth of the muscle groups are the abdominals or the "abs". These muscles are also known as the core and they hold the upper and lower body together. They are a popular muscle group to train as it gives you a flatter stomach or the desired 6 pack of abs.

The abs work together with the back to support and move your torso when you twist to look behind you, or when you bend over to touch your toes. They are also used to keep your organs in place, assist with your breathing and maintain a good posture.

To train your abs you can do:

- Planks

- Crunches

- Sit Ups

Putting It All Together

So now that we have covered the muscle groups and the types of exercises that train each muscle group, let us put together an exercise routine.

When creating your workout plan, try to find balanced workouts. You should ideally have one exercise for each muscle group, and if you would like to focus on a specific muscle group you can spend a few minutes to do an extra set of targeted exercises for that muscle.

Remember that you should do 3 to 5 sets of 10 repetitions for each exercise.

5 Minutes - Warm Up

Start with 5 minutes of warm up exercises to stretch and loosen your muscles. Make sure to stretch each of your major muscle groups.

25 Minutes - Cardio

Choose one of the following cardio activities:

- Running

- Cycling

- Skipping Rope

5 Minutes - Chest

Choose one of the following chest exercises:

- Push ups

- Bench Presses

- Chest Flies

5 Minutes - Back

Choose one of the following back exercises:

- Pull Ups

- Shrugs

- Deadlifts

- Dumbbell Pullovers

- Shoulder Presses

- Barbell Rows

5 Minutes - Arms

Choose one of the following arm exercises:

- Barbell Curls

- Reverse Grip Curls

- Pull Ups

- Bench Presses

- Tricep Extensions

- Dips

- Overhead Presses

- Shoulder Presses

5 Minutes - Legs and Glutes

Choose one of the following leg and glute exercises:

- Squats

- Side Skates

- Hip Thrusts

- Romanian Deadlifts

- Rope Skipping

- Lunges

- Calf Raises

- Ankle Circles

- Balance Boards

5 Minutes - Abs

Choose one of the following abs exercises:

- Planks

- Crunches

- Sit Ups

5 Minutes - Cool Down

End with 5 minutes of cool down activity to release the tension from your muscles. Similar to warming up, be sure to stretch and relax every muscle group.

Remember that you do not have to spend hours to do this, ideally, you should be done in an hour.

CHAPTER 6

Proper Execution of Exercises

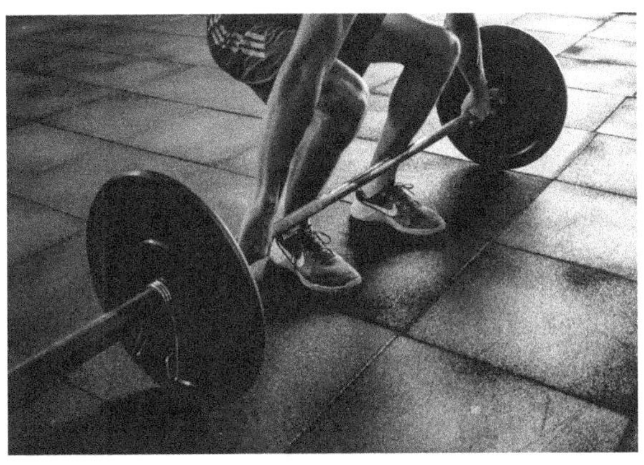

Now that you have your work out plan, you are probably wondering how to do some of the exercises, especially if you are new to the gym. The easiest way is to work with a personal trainer or to watch an exercise video on YouTube. Some of these like running and cycling are pretty straightforward, but for the other exercises that you may not know, I will try to explain here in this chapter.

You may need to use weights or some other equipment for some exercises, which I will mention where necessary. Also, I will let you know if there is anything you need to watch out for as well doing these exercises.

There are also gym machines that you can use to emulate the use of weights. These can be a great substitute for the dumbbell or barbell versions.

1. Push ups

Technique:

- Start with your hands shoulder width apart on the floor and your legs together. Your body should be a straight line supported with only your arms and your toes on the ground.

- Lower your body until your face is nearly touching the ground, then raise your body up using your arms.

2. Bench Presses

Equipment:

- Gym Bench

- Barbell

Technique:

- Lie with your back on the gym bench and grip the barbell with your hands. Your feet should be flat on the ground, or if you prefer you could put them flat on the bench with your knees up.

- Lower the barbell with weights to your chest until it touches your sternum.

- Raise the bar to its original position.

Caution:

- If you are new to this exercise you should use a spotter to help you ensure the exercise is done correctly. There is a danger of you losing control of the bar and having it fall onto your body if your muscles are not able to cope with the weights.

3. Chest Flies

Equipment:

- 2 Dumbbells

- Gym Bench

Technique:

- Lie down on the gym bench with a dumbbell in each hand.

- Extend your arms directly above your chest.

- Lower the dumbbells to the sides in a controlled manner until your arms are extended at the level of your body.

- Raise the dumbbells in a semi circular motion until they are above your chest.

4. Pull Ups

Equipment:

- A pull up bar

Technique:

- Grip the pull up bar and hang freely.

- Pull yourself up until your chin is above the pull up bar.

- Lower yourself back to the starting position.

Caution:

This exercise requires a good amount of upper body strength and is not for beginners. Be careful when you mount/dismount the bar as they can be a few feet in the air.

5. Shrugs

Equipment:

- Barbell

Technique:

- Stand with your feet shoulder width apart and hold the barbell with both hands with your palms facing towards you.

- Raise your shoulders up.

- Return your shoulders to the starting position.

6. Deadlifts

Equipment:

- Barbell

Technique:

- Stand with your feet hip width apart and bend at the hip to grip the bar.

- Lower your hip and flex your knees while looking forward.

- Lift the bar until it is at the level of your hips. You should be pulling your shoulders back as the bar rises above the knee.

- Lower the bar to the starting position.

Caution:

- Lifting too heavy a weight can cause you to drop the weights.

- When doing deadlifts, the lower back is at risk of being injured. Keep your back straight and rigid throughout the lifts.

- If you are unsure of how to perform a deadlift, get a fitness coach to work with you and do not attempt this on your own..

7. **Romanian Deadlifts**

Equipment:

- Barbell

Technique:

- Stand with your feet hip width apart and hold the bar at hip level with your palms face down. Your knees should be slightly bent.

- Lower the bar by moving your hips backwards as far as you can. Keep the bar close to your body at all times and face forward.

- Slowly return to a standing position by moving your hips forward.

Caution:

- Lifting too heavy a weight can cause you to drop the weights.

- When doing deadlifts, the lower back is at risk of being injured. Keep your back straight and rigid throughout the lifts.

- If you are unsure of how to perform a deadlift, get a fitness coach to work with you and do not attempt this on your own..

8. Dumbbell Pullovers

Equipment:

- A dumbbell
- Gym Bench

Technique:

- Lie on the gym bench with your shoulders on the surface. Your feet should be planted firmly on the floor.

- Hold the dumbbell with both hands over your chest and extend your arms outwards above your body. Your hands should both be holding one of the weighted ends of the dumbbell.

- Keep your arms straight and lower the weight in an arc until the dumbbell is behind your head.

- Raise the dumbbell back above your chest.

Caution:

- Always secure the weights to the dumbbell.

- If you are new to this exercise you should use a spotter to help you ensure the exercise is done correctly. There is a danger of you losing control of the bar and having it fall onto your body if your muscles are not able to cope with the weights.

9. Shoulder Presses

Equipment:

- 2 Dumbbells

Technique:

Sit on a bench or chair with back support with your feet firmly planted on the floor.

Raise your dumbbells to ear level with your elbows slightly bent. The dumbbells should be parallel to the floor. Your head should be resting against the back support.

Raise your arms up and touch the dumbbells lightly over your head.

Lower the dumbbells back to ear level.

10. Barbell Rows

Equipment:

- Barbell

Technique:

- Stand with your feet under the bar and bend over to grab the bar with both hands.

- Lift your chest and straighten your back while lifting the weights to shin or ankle height.

- Pull the bar against your chest.

- Lower the bar back to shin or ankle height.

Caution:

- Keep your blower back neutral to avoid back injuries. Do not round or lift with your back.

- Put the bar on the ground between reps if it is too heavy. This will help to prevent injury as well.

11. Barbell Curls

Equipment:

- Barbell

Technique:

- Stand with your back straight and legs about shoulder width apart and hold the barbell in both hands with your elbows close to your body. Your palms should be facing outwards.

- Keep your upper arms and shoulders in place while using your biceps to lift the weights. Only your forearms should be moving.

- Lower the barbell slowly.

12. Reverse Grip Curls

Equipment:

- Barbell

Technique:

This is similar to the barbell curl (above) but you grip with your palms facing your body.

Stand with your back straight and legs about shoulder width apart and hold the barbell in both hands with your elbows close to your body. Your palms should be facing inwards.

Keep your upper arms and shoulders in place while using your biceps to lift the weights. Only your forearms should be moving.

Lower the barbell slowly.

13. Tricep Extensions

Equipment:

- Dumbell

Technique:

- Stand with your feet shoulder width apart and hold a dumbbell with both hands.

- Slowly lift the dumbbell over your head until your arms are fully extended and your palms are facing upwards.

- Keep your elbows close to your head and lower the dumbbell behind your head. Your forearms should touch your biceps when complete.

- Lift the dumbbell over your head with your arms fully extended and your palms face upwards.

14. Dips

Equipment:

- A benche

Technique:

- Position yourself between 2 benches perpendicular to your body.

- Put your hands on the bench behind you and hold the edge of that bench.

- Lower your body slowly by bending your elbows and keep your elbows as close as possible.

- Lift your body back up again.

15. Overhead Presses

Equipment:

- Barbell

Technique:

- Grip the barbell with a wide grip and position the barbell behind your neck and above your shoulders. The bar should not be resting on your body and should only be supported by your hands.

- Keep your elbows under the bar and extend your arms with the barbell overhead.

- Lower the barbell behind your neck and just above your shoulders again.

16. Squats

Equipment:

- Barbell (optional)

Technique:

- Stand with your feet slightly wider than your hips. Point your toes outward.

- If you choose to use a barbell, you should hold it behind your head, above your shoulders. If you are not using a barbell, you should keep your arms straight in front of your body for balance.

- Push your hips backwards as you bend your knees while keeping your back straight and looking forward. Keep squatting until your hips are lower than your knees.

- Reverse the motion and push your hips in while straightening your knees.

17. Side Skates

Technique:

- Stand on a mat in a half squat position.

- Jump sideways to the left side. When you go to the left, land on your left leg and put your right leg behind your left ankle without touching the floor.

- Jump to the right side and land on your right leg. Put your left leg behind your right ankle without touching the floor.

18. Hip Thrusts

Equipment:

- Gym bench

Technique:

- Begin by sitting on the ground with a bench behind. Put your arms on the bench and lean back so your shoulder blades are near the top of the bench.

- Drive your hips upwards using the feet. You may have to tiptoe to get the full motion. You should finish with your body bent only at the knees, and parallel to the ground.

- Relax and lower your body.

19. Lunges

Technique:

- Stand upright with your feet apart and your knees unlocked.

- Take a step forward with one foot and lower the knee of your other leg. Your body should be upright and your knee should be off the ground. The front leg should have its knee bent at a 90 degree angle.

- Push back up with your front foot and step back, bringing your knee of the other leg back beside the other.

- Repeat with the other leg.

20. Calf Raises

Technique:

- Stand with the ball of your feet on the edge of a step. Your heels should be unsupported.

- Raise your heel above the step so that you're on tip toes. You can hold this position for a while if you like.

- Lower your heels back to below the step.

21. Ankle Circles

Technique:

- Steady your body using a wall, chair, or some other object and lift one leg in the air.

- Perform a clockwise motion with your toes, like you are drawing a circle with it.

- Repeat with the other leg.

22. Planks

Technique:

- Lie on the floor and lift your body up. Support your weight using your toes and your forearms. Your elbows should be bent and below your shoulders.

- Keep your body straight at all times and hold this position.

23. Crunches

Technique:

- Lie on your back with your knees bent and your feet firmly on the floor. Put your hands beside your ears or behind your head. Your elbows should be facing outwards.

- Curl up and bring your knees up and your elbows forward at the same time. They do not need to touch.

- Relax and lie back with your knees bent and your feet on the floor.

24. Sit Ups

Technique:

- Lie on your back with your feet secure and your knees bent. Put your hands beside your ears or behind your head. Your elbows should be facing outwards.

- Raise your shoulders and torso towards your knee, ensuring that your elbows touch the knees.

- Relax and go back to lying on your back.

CHAPTER 7

The OMAD Diet

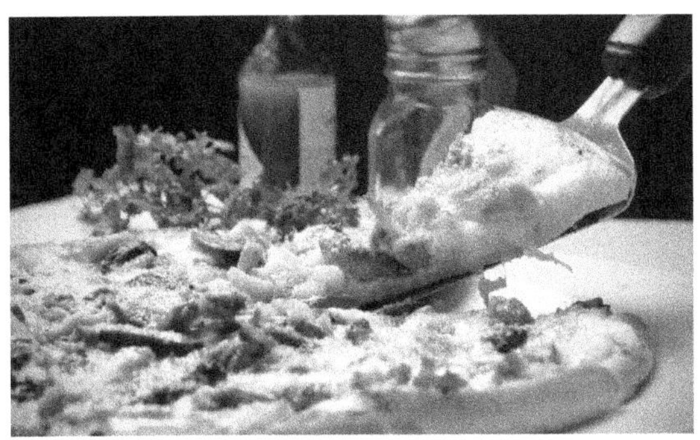

The One Meal a Day (OMAD) Diet is a weight loss method based on intermittent fasting. The main principles of this are regulating your meal frequency, and meal timing. This is a proven way that many people have used to lose body fat and keep it off.

Note that this is not a fad diet, nor is it a temporary weight loss solution.

Most diets are short term and result in a yo-yo effect where people actually lose weight but then they are unable to keep themselves off a pizza or chocolate bar.

They end up caving in to their cravings, or they are unsatisfied with the weight loss that they have achieved. Either way, they end up giving up on their diet and some even gain more weight than they have lost while on a diet.

The issue is that these diets do not address the root cause of weight loss, which is to manage the circadian rhythm. This is done by timing exercise, meals and sleep which is managed when we stick to the rule of 4 "Ones" of the OMAD diet which will be covered in this chapter.

The reason the OMAD diet works is because it is a lifestyle and one that works for the long term because it is based in science. If you can follow the plan you will improve your health, energy, and well being. You do not have to count calories, worry about what you can or cannot eat, and mostly you do not have to feel guilty for cheat days.

Starting the OMAD Diet

While eating one meal a day may sound simple at first, there is a recommended approach to this diet. Like any other diet, the beginning of the switch in eating habits will require conscious effort to maintain, and you will need to build on this consistently in order to achieve long term success. When you are consistent in your daily eating habits, the diet starts to take effect and help you achieve the weight loss that you have set out for yourself.

The basis of the OMAD diet is the rule of 4 "Ones".

In essence, this means you should have:

1. One Hour

2. One Meal

3. One Plate

4. One Beverage

This rule helps you to maintain the discipline and have a structure to your diet. Many people have found this method to work best for weight loss, as well as maintaining a long term healthy lifestyle. So how do you follow the Rule of 4 Ones?

One Hour

When starting the one meal a day diet, you need to choose a four hour window to eat. This can be any four hours you want, but make sure it will best fit into your schedule as it would be best to stay consistent with the eating window.

Once you have chosen your four hour window, you should allow yourself one hour for your meal so you have sufficient time to enjoy your food which can include a beverage of your choice. When the hour is up, there should be no more calorie intake until the next eating window.

When choosing your eating window, it might take some time to figure out how to choose the best one to fit your situation, but maintaining a structure will make all the difference in your weight loss journey.

One Meal

Each day, you will have a 4 hour eating window but you should only give yourself 1 hour in those 4 hours to eat. In that one hour, you will have only one meal.

In the OMAD diet, there should be no small meals or cheat hours where you can eat snacks or junk food.

The only exception to this is for protein shakes taken post workout. If you do workout, these protein shakes are necessary to fuel your body with protein.

One Plate

Since you are restricted to one meal, it may be tempting to pile on whatever you want in your one hour window. When you are eating your one meal, it's important to understand what is going on your plate and ensure that there is a balance of nutrients, proteins, and carbohydrates.

It is recommended to incorporate a serving of vegetables, carbohydrates (potatoes, rice, or bread), protein and fats (from meats), and a serving of fruits.

The caloric intake for most people during OMAD is around 1,500 Kcal.

An average sized plate could actually hold two servings of meals so it is important that you make an informed choice of what goes onto your plate and not overeat during your one meal.

One Beverage

During your meal, you should allow yourself to have one beverage of your choice. This can be anything you crave, from beer to a soda, or anything else you want. This serves as a perk me up to boost your mood. The OMAD diet is not about depriving yourself, it is just a structured way to approach your food and drink intake.

Taking a drink with a caloric count can also help you to get your calories required for the day, but you should keep yourself to one serving.

Apart from this, you should continue to hydrate yourself by drinking water throughout the day. You do not have to limit your intake of water. Tea and coffee can also be drunk at any time, as it may help to suppress your hunger.

What to Expect When Starting OMAD

When starting out on OMAD diets, the most common thing that people experience is hunger, as one would expect, so know that you are not alone. This is most likely an issue of body conditioning that you will have to battle the first few weeks. You may not actually be hungry, but because you have been eating several times a day, your body has been conditioned to expect food every few hours. This is something that everyone on the OMAD diet would have to push through.

While this will vary from person to person, a "fasting headache" is common for the first few weeks at least. This is triggered by a combination of low blood sugar, dehydration, and possibly lack of sleep. The trick is to stay hydrated throughout your fast as it will help to ease the headaches and hunger pangs.

The brain is 75% water and is very sensitive to dehydration, and produced histamines to ration and conserve water when faced with a shortage. It is these histamines that cause headaches as well as fatigues; they are a signal that we need to drink more water. Keep in mind that this discomfort will end once your body gets used to your new eating schedule and the lack of intermittent snacks throughout the day.

Another good way of keeping hunger at bay is to keep yourself busy with work or distracting yourself with other activities. This will help you keep your mind off food. Consciously staying away from the kitchen or the pantry will also help as you will not be constantly seeing and smelling food to whet your appetite when it is not your meal time. Out of sight, out of mind.

Once your mind has been disciplined to eat only meal a day, your body will adjust eventually.

CHAPTER 8

Breaking Your Fast Post Work Out

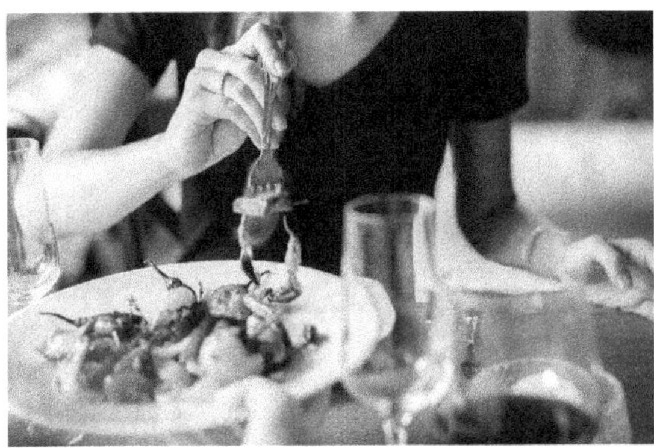

When you are on the OMAD diet, your post workout meals are very important. Since you will be exercising on an empty stomach, there is an anabolic window after your workout. This is when your muscles are receptive to nutrients, and this period lasts anywhere from 1 to 3 hours after your workout. It is therefore very important that you break your fast at most one hour after your workout so you can fuel your body and rebuild your muscles.

What to Eat when Working Out

If you're on the OMAD diet and want to build muscle bulk, a high amount of protein is necessary for muscle synthesis. When we exercise, our muscles are broken down and they need to repair themselves throughout the day. This is how they grow, and protein is necessary for this to happen.

Bodybuilders have a rule of thumb where they take 1 gram of protein per pound of their body weight. When trying to lose fat, some bodybuilders can increase that ratio to 1.5 grams per pound.

Studies have shown that the ratio of protein intake to bodyweight is roughly 0.13% to 0.18%. Meaning that you need about 0.2 - 0.3 ounces of protein for every pound you weigh although other factors such as the intensity and frequency of your workout, your age, and your gender can affect this.

Healthy fats such as nuts, seeds, avocado, cheese, and dark chocolate are also a great source of fuel for your body. Increasing your intake of healthy fats also helps to decrease cravings, which would prevent you from going hungry after exercising.

Aside from proteins, carbohydrates are another important part of our diet. It is recommended that we eat whole-grain cereals (with low-fat or skim milk), whole-wheat toast, low-fat or fat-free yogurt, whole grain pasta, brown rice, fruits, and vegetables when working out on the OMAD diet. These are more complex carbohydrates that take longer to be digested, and help to stave off hunger as well as reduce the spikes in our blood glucose.

Sugars and grains are also carbohydrates but should be avoided as much as possible along with processed food. These foods cause cravings as well as our blood sugar to spike severely which overworks our body's digestive system. After the "sugar rush" also comes a crash in blood sugar which brings about hunger and the craving for more food.

Remember that our bodies are different, and we all adjust to routines differently. When making any changes to habits, introduce them slowly and give it some time to take effect and show results otherwise it will lead to frustration.

The important thing is that we are consistent with our diet, our eating window, and our workout routine as the OMAD diet is a lifestyle.

Also, you must remember to hydrate yourself before and after your work outs. This has been mentioned several times in this book, but the effects of dehydration can be severe. Exercising while dehydrated has been linked to kidney failure, seizures, and even death.

When Should You Eat? Post or Pre Workout

When you are trying to build muscles you will need to provide your body with protein and amino acids. These are the building blocks of your muscles which you will need to repair the muscles and enable them to grow after exercise.

Post work out, it is important that you break your fast and get nutrients to your muscle cells as fast as possible. When you elevate your insulin levels it will help to drive nutrients to your cells.

In this situation, carbohydrates are especially important as they are depleted when you exercise and need to be replaced. High protein foods like red meat are also necessary as they will easily satisfy your body's requirements for nutrients as they are easily assimilated into the cells of your muscles. Lastly, you might also want to consider adding healthy fats such as avocado, cheese, or fatty fish. These healthy fats help to keep your blood sugar more stable and do not cause an insulin response in your body so including some healthy fats in your meals will help to decrease food cravings.

This would be an ideal post workout meal to break your fast.

While the post-workout meal is important, it is also essential for you to consider pre-workout meals as sometimes you will need to work out after your meal or you may feel less dizzy and fatigued if you eat something before your work out. If you choose to exercise after your meal you should still consume something like a high protein or high (healthy) snack after your exercise.

Note that this is not strictly OMAD, but remember that we all have our individual physiologies so you should do what works best for you. If you feel unwell or uncomfortable at any time during your fast, you should stop fasting and try again once you feel better.

A pre workout meal or snack will help to stimulate protein synthesis when you are exercising. This will prevent muscle breakdown when you are exercising. A study conducted in 2014 found that fasting for at least 10 hours puts the body in fat metabolism while avoiding muscle catabolism at the same time. When you eat before exercise, especially if you are planning a high intensity workout, it gives your body the energy it needs.

Planning your meal pre or post workout is crucial when on OMAD. You can opt not to have a pre workout meal but you should never skip the post workout meal, even if it's just a snack.

For most people, a 20 gram protein bar or shake before working out can help with fat burning as well as promote muscle growth. Remember that you are trying to lose fat and gain or maintain your muscles, not lose it. Other options are to eat some Greek yogurt with berries or nuts, hard boiled eggs, or a low carb granola bar.

The most important thing when deciding your approach is to listen to your body. If you feel weak or dizzy when exercising on an empty stomach, stop your exercise and eat something. Your health and well being should be your priority, and your body will adjust to your fasting and exercise routine over time.

Principles When Planning Your Post-Workout Meals

There are several things to consider when you are planning your post workout meals in order to get the most benefit out of it. Below are some guidelines I use when I am planning my meals and exercise routines.

1. Fast for at least 20 hours daily.

2. Strictly eat within the 4-hour feeding window.

3. Exercise with a high intensity workout twice week while in a fasted state.

4. Consume at least 10 grams of protein before exercising.

5. During your exercise days, consume a meal comprised of protein, vegetables, and small amounts of carbohydrates.

6. During non-exercise days, eat a meal of protein, vegetables, and fats. Consume only whole and minimally-processed foods.

While this may not suit everyone due to our personal preferences, different physiologies, and individual schedules you can use this as a starting point and adjust them to your needs.

Maybe you need to have a larger feeding window, or you may require more protein before your work out. Try it out, adjust what doesn't work, and adopt what works best for you.

CHAPTER 9

Nutrition on OMAD and Exercise

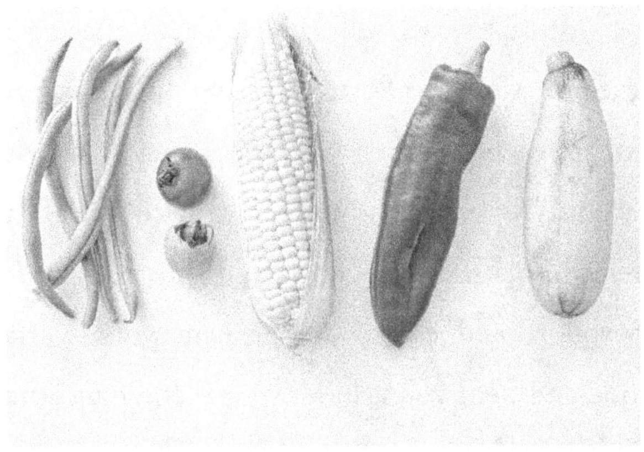

Now that we have discussed when to eat your meals, in this chapter we will be looking at what to eat during your meals. While when we eat is important on the OMAD diet, what we eat determines how we look and feel. After all, it is commonly said that "we are what we eat".

There are many studies on nutrition when exercising and they all point to the fact that the food we choose to eat is just as important as exercise if not more important than exercise. A well balanced meal is an important part of a healthy lifestyle, especially when combined with exercise.

The 3 Main Nutrients

The foods that we eat will have different effects when we exercise while in a fasted state. Our bodies will have different reactions when we have a huge amount of carbs and not enough protein or vice versa. It is therefore important to understand the types of food that you should eat to complement your workout routine and help you achieve your dieting and fitness goals.

Carbohydrates

Carbohydrates are found in almost all foods and provide 4 calories of energy per gram. Foods that contain carbs basically fall into two types:

1. Simple Carbohydrates:

These are also called sugars and are made from glucose, fructose, and galactose. Because the chains of these carbohydrate molecules are short they are easier to break down and are easily digested and absorbed into the bloodstream.

Foods such as sugar, honey, jellies, jams, as well as products made from flour like white bread and cake contain simple carbohydrates.

2. Complex Carbohydrates:

Complex carbohydrates come in two forms and are either a starch or a fibre. While they are made up of the same sugars as simple carbs, complex carbs have an additional sugar molecule with a longer chain. This makes complex carbs more difficult to break down and digest. This slows down the absorption into the bloodstream, which prevents insulin levels from spiking.

Brown rice, wheat and wholemeal bread, beans, and vegetables are all examples of complex carbohydrates as are bananas and berries.

When you are on OMAD, it is beneficial for you to choose complex carbohydrates, especially those that contain high fibre. Vegetables and whole grain are examples of high fibre complex carbohydrates. Since they take longer to break down in your body, these will keep you full for a longer time and also prevent spikes in your blood sugar.

When on exercise you should take some carbs, it is after all the preferred fuel source for your body. Carbs are what fuels your workouts, although if you overload on carbs and do not burn off the excess calories they will be stored as fat in your body. One of the reasons we are seeing more obese people is because their calorie consumption is higher than their energy output.

When choosing **carbohydrates** you should consider:

- Whole grains

- Oatmeal

- Brown rice

- Sweet potatoes

- Bananas

- Pears

- Apples

- Oranges

Protein

Protein is a key component of every single cell in our bodies. They are made up of amino acids which are essential for growth and the repair of broken down tissue - which is the result of exercise. Additionally, the amino acids found in protein cannot be produced by our own bodies. Since our bodies cannot produce its own protein, they must be supplied by our the food we eat.

When we do not have enough protein, our bodies are put in a catabolic state where it tears down our muscle tissue to meet its protein needs.

While protein is also a source of energy like carbs and fat, it has many other functions as well, and it cannot be converted into fat and stored in our bodies like carbs. For that reason, the body digests carbohydrates and fat first before protein to get energy.

That is why we need to eat protein when working out. We want to lose fat and gain muscle, and not the other way around.

When choosing protein, a lean cut of beef or pork like tenderloin or chuck can reduce the calories you gain from fat. Plat based protein, fish, or poultry are also good alternatives.

When choosing **proteins** you should consider:

- Lean beef

- Chicken

- Turkey

- Fish

- Eggs

- Low fat dairy

Fat

Fat has an undeserved reputation. There is a common belief that eating fat makes you... fat. However, fat is not always a bad thing as it has many benefits aside from just making your food taste good. Fats are a very dense source of energy, holding 9 calories per gram. That is more than double what you get from carbohydrates.

In addition, fat can contain many nutrients such as essential fatty acids such as omega-3 and omega-6 which support your nerves and respond to inflammation. Fats also contain cholesterol which is used to keep your cells healthy. Note that too much cholesterol can lead to heart disease, and if you lack this in your diet your body can manufacture the cholesterol it needs. Lastly, fats also contain vitamins. Notably, vitamins A, D, E, and K.

Fats are composed of building blocks called fatty acids, which fall into four main categories:

1. **Polyunsaturated**

   Polyunsaturated fat are also found in animal and plant oils. These are healthy oils and can lower your LDL cholesterol (bad cholesterol) levels. These include omega-3 and omega-9 acids that is needed for brain and cell function. Note that polyunsaturated fat is not produced by our bodies.

   While polyunsaturated fat is consider healthy, it should also be consumed in moderation. If reducing your blood cholesterol is a health goal, eliminating saturated fats is much more effective than increasing your consumption of polyunsaturated fats.

Polyunsaturated fat can be found in corn oil, sunflower oil, fatty fish, flax seeds, and walnuts.

2. Monounsaturated

Monounsaturated fat is found exclusively in plant foods such as olives, nuts, avacados, and vegetable oils. These are also healthy fats that can help lower your LDL cholesterol, similar to polyunsaturated fat.

A way to tell the "healthy" fats apart from "unhealthy" fats is that Saturated fats and trans fats are in a solid state when at room temperature. Monounsaturated fat and polyunsaturated fat are in a liquid state at room temperature, but will harden to a solid when chilled.

3. Saturated

Saturated fats are found in animal and dairy products as well as some plant based oils. Saturated fats when consumed can be processed by the liver to make cholesterol which is then used to produce hormones in our bodies. Consuming some fat in our diet helps to keep our body's hormone levels up at optimal levels.

Foods that have saturated fat are: whole milk, cheese, red meat, coconut oil, and vegetable shortening.

4. Trans Fats

Of all the types of fats, trans fat is the worst of the lot. Too much trans fat poses a risk for heart disease, but we need to understand the difference between naturally occurring trans fat, and the processed trans fat.

Natural trans fat can be found in some meat and dairy products such as beef and lamb. These are less of a concern if you choose low fat or lean cuts.

Processed trans fats occur when polyunsaturated fat such as vegetable oil is made into a solid like margarine through a chemical process called hydrogenation. This changes the physical properties of the fat such as the melting point, which is desirable when mixing with flour for baking. However this has a side effect on our health and can manifest as circulatory or heart disease.

Thankfully, the food industry are moving away from processed trans fats and using other sources of fat in our food. Trans fats are also frequently found in labels on food packaging.

In general, fat intake should be kept low when you are working out and trying to put on muscle. In fact, many bodybuilders practice eating "clean". That is sticking mainly to lean meats, dairy, and complex carbohydrates, with the option of adding supplements of omega-3 to get their recommended dosage of healthy fat.

Most foods are a combination of all saturated, unsaturated, and monounsaturated fat, although one is typically the dominant type which therefore dictates it's classification.

When choosing **fats** you should consider:

- Flaxseed

- Sunflower seeds

- Canola oil

- Olive oil

When choosing **fats** you should avoid or reduce:

- Processed vegetable oils

- Butter

- Lard

- Margarine

The Nutrient Ratio You Need for Weight Loss

When we are trying to lose weight through diet and exercise, we want to not only need to output more calories than we take in, we would also need to make smart choices on what to eat and what not to eat in order to achieve our goals. This will help us to reduce our fat and replace it with muscle which helps to set our bodies up for a higher resting metabolism. This means that our bodies will burn more calories while at rest when we have more muscles.

As we learned in the earlier part of this chapter, carbs are an important source of fuel for our muscles and it is also the only source of energy for our brain and red blood cells. Fat helps with brain function and cell development. Lastly, protein is used to build and repair muscle tissue. Therefore, not all foods are equal. We want to consider how much of these 3 nutrients we want to take in order to support our goals.

When you are on OMAD there are additional considerations because your feeding window is very small. You will need to make the right food choices to get the most nutritional value in your one meal and keep in mind the rule of 4 "ones". With your one plate you should be aiming for 1,500 calories- 2,000 calories for men, and between 1,200 calories - 1,500 calories for women.

Protein is necessary, and arguably the most important component of an OMAD diet. The recommended dietary allowance for protein is 0.36 grams per pound of bodyweight. That means for an average person who weighs about 165 pounds, you will need 60 grams of protein per day. However, when you are exercising you will need more. For an average person again, the protein intake should be easily doubled. Cutting down on protein means that you won't get enough amino acids which will put you in a catabolic state, causing you to ultimately lose lean muscle.

Fats in our diet are just as equally important as they regulate your hormones and your thyroid. The recommended daily allowance of fat is 15% of your daily calories but on OMAD it is recommended that you increase this to at least 20% which is about 40 grams of fat on a 2,000 calorie diet. If you are going low carb, or even keto it should be even higher. Some people have managed to maintain a diet of up to 150 grams of fat and stay healthy. Just remember to choose healthy, polyunsaturated or monounsaturated fats.

Carbohydrates are the least important of the three nutrients. While the recommended daily allowance for carbs is 50%, restricting carbs often have a positive effect on weight loss. When choosing your carbs, you should make healthier choices as far as possible.

Remember that this fruits such as apples, bananas, berries, and vegetables all have carbs but they are all healthy choices as they contain vitamins, fiber, and other nutrients. If you choose to have pasta, rice, bread, or other flour bread products a multigrain option is more beneficial for you.

If you exercise often and have an active lifestyle, then having more carbs in your diet may not be a bad thing. Still, you can do OMAD with minimal carbs or without carbs at all, but it is not optimal as you will be missing out on a lot of vegetables, fruits, and other plant based foods. While you can survive on a zero-carb diet it should ultimately be your personal choice.

Lastly, there is no magic ratio for everyone. The optimal ratio is largely dependent on our individual physiologies and whether there are any health problems like type 2 diabetes or problems with our metabolism. The beautiful thing, however, is that on the OMAD diet you don't really need to obsess over this. It is certainly good to keep in mind your ratio of protein to fat to carbs but most of all you should enjoy the foods you eat and make a conscious choice to eat healthily and enjoy your meals. When you have a healthy relationship with food it will definitely impact your health and weight in a positive manner.

CHAPTER 10

Supplements While Working Out on OMAD

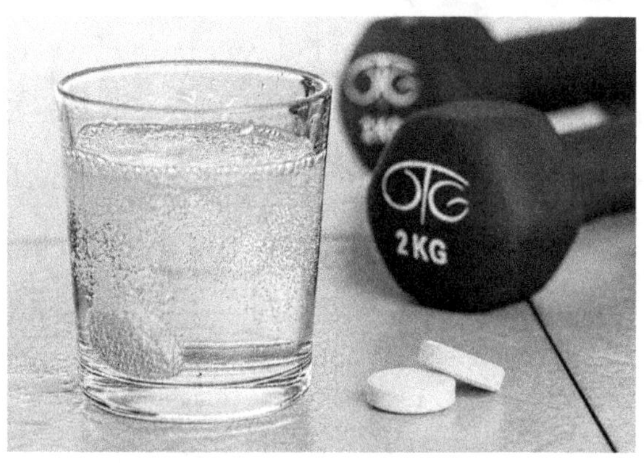

Our bodies need a certain amount of essential vitamins and minerals to function, and many people will tell you that you should supplement your meals when fasting. However, the truth is that you don't need to have a constant stream of vitamins in your body.

Most of your minerals are stored in your bones, fat, liver, and other places. When you fast, your body will break down and catabloze the dead cells and start to use up the nutrients that are stored up. However, this only occurs if you fast for long periods of over 48 hours.

Just to be clear, you do not need to take any supplements on OMAD.

Choosing to take supplements, however, is another issue. If you are on a high protein, high fat diet, then having some supplements can help you balance your meals and achieve better overall health. Some supplements can also help when you are fasting and working out. Consuming these would definitely help you maintain your fast and get the most benefit from your exercise.

With supplements, you need to consider your medical condition, metabolism, and the type of supplements you want to take. It is best to check with a pharmacist or a doctor, especially if you are on any medication when adding supplements.

BCAAs

First let's get one thing clear about Branched Chain Amino Acids (BCAA): They will break your fast.

So what are BCAAs? They are an amino acid with a different "branched" structure of carbons that allow our bodies to transport BCAAs from the liver to the bloodstream directly.

BCAAs are supplements that contain amino acids, which are the building blocks of protein. They help keep our muscles in a non-catabolic state and also help support endurance while working out as well as improve the muscle recovery.

But more than boosting the endurance and building muscles, amino acid supplements also reduce fatigue, increase fat loss, and also improve the cognitive function of the brain. Moreover, it also has anti-inflammatory properties and can remove inflammation on the joints and muscles.

There are 9 amino acids in total, but the main ones that BCAAs contain are Valine, Leucine, and Isoleucine.

BCAAs have a caloric value of 6 Cal per gram and will trigger an insulin response in our bodies because they contain proteins. Since fasting is meant to keep your insulin levels low, taking BCAAs will break your fast.

BCAAs are present in the food we eat and you can get them if you eat foods such as whey, casein protein shakes, eggs, beef, chicken, and fish.

Taking BCAAs are said to protect against muscle loss. However, they've been shown to be effective only if you exercise in a fasted state. Taking BCAAs while fasting will also give you extra energy, and if you are pushing yourself during your work out you may be able to perform better and get more fat loss or muscle gain.

Casein Protein Powder

Similar to BCAAs, casein will also break your fast.

Casein is a slow digesting dairy protein consisting of 80% milk protein. This means that it feeds your cells with amino acids over a long period of time.

A lesser known fact about casein is that it helps to synthesize protein, even when your body might be breaking down its own muscles. This happens when fasting, and it makes casein beneficial for an OMAD diet as the slower digestive process keeps the amino acids in your body longer.

In addition to the above, there are some more benefits found in research on casein:

- **Antibacterial and immune benefits:** casein may provide antibacterial and immune benefits as well as reduce high blood pressure.

- **Fat loss:** fat loss is improved by three times when on casein

- **Reduction in free radicals:** peptides in casein protein powder may have antioxidant effects.

- **Triglyceride levels:** casein reduced triglyceride levels after a meal by 22%.

Creatine

Creatine monohydrate is a performance enhancing supplement that is popular among athletes and bodybuilders. It can improve your cells' ability to produce Adenosine Triphosphate (ATP) which provides energy for your muscles. It is believed to improve strength, increase muscle growth, and help muscles recover during exercise. This is especially so during short periods of intense activity such as weight lifting.

So what happens when you take creatine when fasting?

Unlike casein and BCAAs, creatine will not break your fast as it does not contain calories. In fact, it is popular with people who practice fasting in one form or another.

However, to get the full effects of creatine you will need to combine the effects of creatine with insulin as it will produce greater results. Creatine acts as a buffer for liquid retention and inhibits fluid absorption. That means that your muscle holds more water which will impact your muscle performance when insulin and creatine are present in your body at the same time. In a fasted state, creatine is still absorbed but it will take more time.

If you do want to take creatine, you should take it with your meals and workouts. Creatine doses of 5 grams daily are more than enough to reap the benefits and improve your physical performance and help you build muscle.

Multivitamins

Multivitamins provide the necessary elements so that your body can carry out different physiological functions. When you are on the OMAD diet, you may want to supplement your meal with a multivitamin that provides you with your daily requirements of vitamins. As you are only eating one plate of food it may not be possible to get everything on that one plate all the time.

Multivitamins are a sure way to get your daily requirements of vitamins and minerals that your body needs.

Some vitamins are easier to absorb with food, while others work fine when fasted. When you take vitamins on an OMAD diet you will need to experiment with what works best for you. If you feel dizzy or weak when you take your vitamins you may need to change your schedule.

If they upset your stomach or make you feel dizzy, you may need to moderate them. You should pay attention to how you feel and how your body reacts to the multivitamins you are taking. Over time, you should find out what works best for you.

Healthy Fats

While there are many types of fat supplements on the market, the main supplement is fish oil which contains high amounts of omega-3 fatty acids. Fish oil comes from the tissue of cold water fishes as they generally have a higher fat content.

Examples of these fish are salmon, anchovies, sardines, and tuna.

Taking a fish oil supplement helps to improve our blood pressure, blood lipids, and heart rate. Aside from the cardiovascular benefits, It also serves as an anti-inflammatory agent. These findings are from a study published by the Mayo Clinic in 2017.

When choosing a fish oil to take, you should look out for one that is purified and free of heavy metals and other harmful toxins.

L-Carnitine

L-carnitine is a naturally synthesized amino acid that is produced in our bodies when we burn fat and remove toxins in the cells. Since it is naturally produced and our bodies make enough for our needs we would almost never encounter a deficiency in this compound unless we have a medical disorder or are on some medication, usually kidney disease.

There are claims that L-carnitine can help with fatigue, improve athletic performance, and improve heart health. However, all of these currently lack sufficient evidence as the research is still in the early stages. Despite what many others may claim, this is not backed up by science at the moment.

There are very likely no side effects from taking L-carnitine, but just as likely no benefit to most people.

If you wish to take this supplement, I would recommend discussing with your doctor first.

Vitamin D

This is a fat soluble vitamin that helps your body to absorb calcium and phosphorus which is important for your bone health and can prevent osteoporosis. It can be made by our bodies when our skin is exposed to sunlight which includes vitamins D1, D2, and D3. As a supplement, vitamin D is best taken after food although it can be taken on an empty stomach as well.

A study by the British Journal of Nutrition in 2008 has linked vitamin D supplementation with fat loss and proposed a link with a calcium specific appetite control for obese women.

In 2011, a group of German researchers published a paper on PubMed that links vitamin D supplementation to the testosterone levels in men. Vitamin D was found to benefit the male reproductive tract and have a positive effect on the prostate.

Iodine

Iodine is a supplement that is needed in our bodies. We usually get it from our food intake since this cannot be naturally produced, but there is very little iodine in food unless it has been added during processing. Sea kelp, or seaweed, is the best known source of iodine, but strawberries, eggs, and yogurts contain some as well. However, if you need to supplement iodine it is best that you take it in the form of capsules.

While on the OMAD diet, there is no additional reason to supplement iodine in our diets other than the fact that iodine deficiency is a common health issue worldwide.

CHAPTER 11

Myths on Nutrition, Exercise, and Fasting

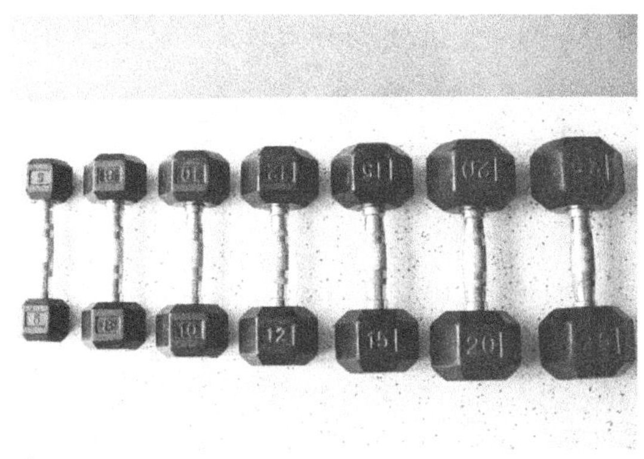

Mainstream nutrition is filled with myths and half truths usually passed down from old wives tales and folk wisdom. Even in this day and age as nutrition science advances, I am still amazed by the beliefs that some people have on nutrition. Now add fasting into the mix, and that adds a whole dimension to the myths.

However, when you are serious about getting in shape false beliefs and bad information can do harm to your body. It pays to be informed with the facts so here are some of the myths that you need to know about nutrition, fasting, and exercise.

Myth: Our body cannot absorb more than 30 grams of protein

One of the most common myths on protein is that our bodies cannot absorb more than 30 grams at a time.

It has been shown in a 1999 study published in the American Journal of Physiology that consuming protein in excess of 40 grams after exercise can stimulate muscle growth. Consuming a high amount of protein helps to stimulate muscle growth and reduce muscle loss and nowadays many athletes and bodybuilders around the world have adopted this practice.

It has also been found in other studies that if you consume more protein than your body needs, the rest will just be excreted the next time you go to the toilet. Your body will store and take up the amino acids and use it where it is needed by the body and the rest is disposed.

While you may consume more than 30 grams of protein on a meal especially on OMAD, it is not something that you should worry about.

Myth: Cutting carbs will make you skinny

A low carb diet has been a well established method for quick weight loss, but this can actually backfire. When you cut carbs from your diet your body goes into an energy deficit.

When this happens, it can have an effect on your energy, mood, appetite, and gut function in the long term. A low carb diet is one which often results in yo-yo dieting as people make up for the lack of energy during the day by overeating.

In fact, cutting carbs causes weight loss through losing water instead of fat. Carbs support the thyroid glad and can assist in providing energy when exercising. So instead of cutting carbs, it is recommended to choose complex carbs or fruit and vegetables as a healthy carb option.

Myth: Eating carbs makes you fat

Carbohydrates serve and important function such as replenishing your body's stores of glycogen. It also helps you to feel full and according to a 2002 study, carbs are also responsible for improving the quality of your sleep.

While our bodies need carbs we need to take it in the right amount and from the right sources. Healthy carbs, such as whole grains, vegetables, fruits, and other complex carbohydrates taken in moderation is a good thing.

Of course you can choose to go low carb or remove them from your diet altogether (with the support of a nutritionist or a doctor) but it is not mandatory for weight loss.

Myth: Eating fat makes you fat

Fat contains more calories per gram compared to carbs and proteins. This gives it the reputation of causing weight gain. What people fail to realize is that fats are a necessary part of our diets just like carbs and proteins.

They all do their part to keep our bodies healthy and they all play a role in our physiologies.

Foods that are high in healthy fats have higher calories and they help to keep us full for a longer period. This helps to control our cravings as there is no insulin spike which means that we do not experience a sugar crash.

It is important that we eat the right fats in the right portions and take a balanced approach to nutrition.

Myth: You can eat as much as you want and whatever you want when you break your fast

The OMAD diet has the rule of 4 "ones", and one of them is restricting you to one plate of food.

This does not mean that you can stack the pizzas on your plate until it starts to fall over. The idea of having one plate is to restrict your portion while ensuring that you have a balance of proteins, fats, and carbs. An average sized plate could actually hold up to two servings of meals therefore you need to make an informed choice of what goes onto your plate.

You should not overeat just because you only have one meal as tempting as it may be.

Additionally, it is recommended to incorporate a serving of vegetables, carbohydrates (potatoes, rice, or bread), protein and fats (from meats), and a serving of fruits. You should aim for a caloric intake around 1,500 Kcal. The key to successfully losing weight on the OMAD diet is to eat normally when breaking your fast. Eating 3 meals in 1 negates the time you spent fasting.

Myth: The longer you spend working out the better

This is the myth that quantity can replace quality, and this myth has been around for a long time. It may seem obvious that the more time you spend working out, the more your muscles will grow.

However, what is more important than the length of your workout is using the right technique and the right intensity for your fitness level. If you have a clear objective with your training you can easily get your workout done in an hour.

This is supported by a paper in the American Physiological Society, published in 2007. It was found that repetitions of shorter exercise can help to metabolize more fat. Breaking a work out into smaller work outs with a rest period in between was found to be more beneficial.

The American College of Sports Medicine has also recommended that the exercise duration should be between 45 minutes to 60 minutes.

Myth: Eating OMAD causes muscle loss

There is a belief that when we fast our body will start to use our fat as fuel. While this happens with any diet, there is no evidence to suggest that it happens more with OMAD or any intermittent fasting diet as compared to other diets.

A study published in the Obesity Reviews in 2011 found that an intermittent caloric restriction caused the same amount of weight loss as a continuous caloric restriction, but with reduced loss in muscle mass.

Another study published by the American Journal of Clinical Nutrition found that eating one huge meal in the evening with the same amount of calories they were used to will actually help people lose body fat and increase muscle mass.

This means that having One Meal A Day is actually more beneficial than other diets with regards to minimizing muscle loss. In addition to that there are additional benefits to fat loss and other health markers.

Myth: Eating one meal a day is bad for your health

A study conducted by the National Institute of Aging concluded eating one meal a day rather than three, decreases your insulin resistance and helps your glucose intolerance. These are both features that are related to type 2 diabetes.

OMAD actually enhances your body's hormone function to facilitate weight loss. When you fast your body adjusts by having lower insulin levels, higher growth hormone levels and increased amounts of norepinephrine. These all help to increase the breakdown of body fat which is then converted into energy.

The American Journal of Clinical Nutrition found that fasting actually increases your metabolic rate by 3.6% to 14%, which helps you burn even more calories.

There are also many other studies that correlate fasting with a longer life spans and improved health.

Myth: Eating OMAD will make you gain weight

While a big meal may have a correspondingly huge amount of calories, you will be in a calorie deficit while fasting. Eating a big meal does not change that as your body will be burning more calories than you take in.

Additionally, research has shown that eating a big meal before you start fasting can preserve muscle mass better when compared to other diets. As long as you stick to the rule of 4 "ones" you will not put on weight by following the OMAD diet.

Myth: Fasting will slow your metabolism down

Since you are eating less often when you fast, it is a common fear that your metabolism will slow down when on OMAD. This is a common myth that has been debunked by the Journal of the Academy of Nutrition and Dietetics in 2015.

The American Journal of Clinical Nutrition have shown in studies that fasting for 48 hours will improve your metabolism by up to 14%, but longer fast will slow your metabolism. Also, fasting on alternate days for a 22 day period does not decrease your metabolic rate but may cause you to lose 4% of body fat.

Remember that the OMAD diet is not about calorie restriction and it is not about denial of your favorite foods, it is about restricting the time in which your body gets its calories.

Myth: I should eat my meal in the morning/afternoon/evening

On the OMAD diet, you can eat your meal anytime that you wish during the day.

There isn't a best or optimal time during the day when eating one meal a day so you should consume your meal whenever it is most convenient for you. Consistency is the key to getting the best results on OMAD. We recommend choosing an eating window that best fits your lifestyle and schedule.

If you are exercising, it is alright to have a snack before your work out if you need to and then break your fast 30 minutes after exercise. Alternatively, you could have your meal first then exercise an hour after that. If you do this, you may want to have some protein after to help your muscles grow.

The only suggestion would be that you leave a few hours after your meal to digest your food before going to bed as it will make you feel less uncomfortable.

Myth: Fasting for 20+ hours a day and eating one meal will give me gastrointestinal distress

We all know that our stomachs have acids to digest and break down our food, and it is a misconception that when there is no food our stomachs will devour itself.

When there is no food in our stomachs the epithelial cells will start to secret mucus and bicarbonate to protect itself and become less acidic in the process. It will adapt to having less food or no food.

Since you are eating only one meal a day, your digestive system isn't as overworked as before. If you reduce highly processed and fatty foods, digestive issues will be reduced even further. Your gut microbes get more diverse and you increase the tolerance against bad microbes which will reduce inflammation of the gut.

If you have gastrointestinal issues the OMAD diet can help because you will not constantly be trying to process food in your gut.

Eating OMAD improves your gastrointestinal health.

Myth: OMAD will negatively impact my mood and energy levels due to hunger

When we fast two things start to happen to our bodies.

Firstly, fasting increases the growth and development of brain cells and nerve tissues. Dr Mark Mattson, a Neurology Professor at John Hopkins University has found that fasting increases the growth and development of brain cells and nerve tissues. Additionally, fasting has also shown to reduce inflammation in the brain which can lead to Alzheimer's and other neurodegenerative disorders.

Secondly, our bodies learn to look for alternate sources of energy such as our fat stores. When we eat once a day our metabolism also changes and our bodies start to use fat instead of food as energy. As fat is slowly digested and sent to the liver for processing it happens steadily over a longer period of time and does not cause spikes in our blood sugar and has less effect on our metabolism.

This is in line with what other people who fast have reported in terms of increased concentration, and better memory. This also results in being more mentally stable and alert during daily tasks.

Myth: All diets restrict calories and OMAD is the same

The daily caloric intake for men is roughly 2,500 kcal and for women 2,000 kcal.

However on OMAD you do not have to count your calories as long as you stick to the rule of 4 "ones". The structure of the 4 "ones" ensures that you will get sufficient calories without overeating, but also allowing you the luxury of your favorite foods.

You can eat until you are feeling full, but know that you will get hungry around your regular eating times. At the start this can be tough, but a good way to gauge is to drink some water and wait for an hour or two. If you're still feeling hungry, then consider breaking your fast.

If you are tracking what you eat for building muscle, then tracking your macros is a totally different issue.

Myth: I will be constantly hungry on the OMAD diet

This is a very common question and usually the first to come up when I mention that I only eat once a day.

The thing is, when you are on the OMAD diet it will become easier the longer you stick to it.

Your body is used to eating three times a day, and maybe with snacks in between, and it has learned to expect food at certain times. The hormone known as ghrelin is responsible for making us feel hunger, and has been found to peak around meal times.

When you fast you can expect ghrelin levels to continue to peak around meal times, especially during the first week. This eventually will pass as your body adapts to your new routine. There are some people who have reported that during their meal windows, they don't even feel hungry. You should give your body time to adapt accordingly as it will take you some time to get used to OMAD.

When starting a fast, drinking water will help to combat the hunger. Some nutritionists explain that the hunger may be dehydration or boredom as eating three times a day is a habit that we have been conditioned with all our lives. Drinking unsweetened coffee and tea may also help with hunger similar to drinking water.

When you are first starting out, it can be tough, but keeping a positive and disciplined mindset will help you achieve success in your diet. Everyone is different as to when your body will adapt to your new lifestyle.

It is alright if you do not follow the OMAD diet every day, you can and should break your fast if you feel unwell, dizzy, or if it is interfering with your daily lifestyle. You can always try again when you feel better.

As with any diet, it's a marathon and not a sprint. Although it is called a "diet", OMAD is actually a lifestyle change and brings with it many benefits.

Discipline is a huge factor in succeeding with the OMAD diet, and it can be difficult at times to deal with the discomfort and the hunger, especially in the initial stages. If you have to break your fast early or take more than one meal it is okay.

This is a long term thing, and it takes time for your body to adapt. There are many people who have tried OMAD and failed many times before succeeding.

Some of them do OMAD only once a week or on alternate days.

To be successful, you just have to stick with it and don't give up. Once you start to see the benefits that self discipline has brought you, you will be more determined to push forward and get the success you wanted.

Conclusion

Thank you for taking the time to read this book!

By now I hope that you have taken action on your fitness or diet routine at least. Once you put the information here to use, your physique will improve along with your health and fitness. Exercise and OMAD together will have tremendous effects, but even if you adopt only one of them you should still see a result that you would be satisfied with.

The next step here is to consult with your doctor and a fitness instructor, begin planning your meals and workouts, and starting on your journey. If you can, take action today; the longer you put things off the more likely you are to continue procrastinating.

Set your goals, adjust your mindset, and take action.

If you have enjoyed this book and want to learn more, please do have a look at my other book on the OMAD diet.

Train safe, eat healthy, and enjoy your meals!

www.ingramcontent.com/pod-product-compliance
Lightning Source LLC
Chambersburg PA
CBHW061350250726
48657CB00004B/1420